THE MIRACLE OF PROPOLIS

THIS BOOK BELONGS
TO JILL CAHMANN

PLEASE RETURN

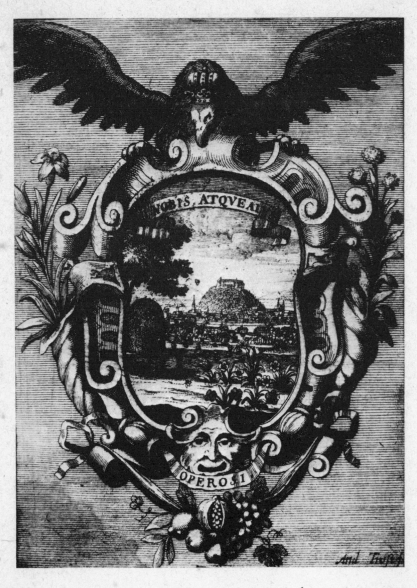

The coat of arms of the *Academia Operosorum*, established in 1701

THE MIRACLE OF PROPOLIS

The Story of the Rediscovery of the
Remarkable Healing Properties of this
Product of the Beehives

by

MITJA VOSNJAK

THORSONS PUBLISHERS LIMITED
Wellingborough, Northamptonshire

First published 1978

ISBN 0 7225 0408 X

Typeset by Specialised Offset Services Ltd., Liverpool
and printed and bound in Great Britain by
Biddles Ltd., Guildford, Surrey

Contents

CHAPTER ONE

A GATHERING OF BEEKEEPERS

In the year 1776 the first written report about propolis appeared. Anton Jansha, from Breznica in northern Slovenia, who was famous as the first person to teach that it is not necessary to kill the bees in order to take their honey, wrote in his book *Complete Instructions for Beekeeping*:

'Another sort of wax is also found which is used by the bees for filling in and plastering over the pores, crevices and cracks in the hive. It is called putty-wax.'

More than half a century later, in the year 1831, linguist and beekeeper Peter Dajnko asked:

'What else do the bees need for their work? A putty or similar substance. They bring it from the wild chestnut, poplar or other trees.'

Then there was silence for a long time.

My story of propolis begins in the village of Repnje, nestled at the foot of the wooded hills near Ljubljana. In front of every home in the village stands a beehive, for in Jugoslavia, perhaps more than in any other country, there is a strong tradition of beekeeping. Here, and nowhere else, there developed during the eighteenth and nineteenth centuries the very beautiful art of painting beehives. The painters created hundreds of small, precious works of art in living colour, which specialists today might perhaps equate with the naïve school of painting.

The bee also became the symbol of progress in science and culture in Jugoslavia. In 1701 the first scientific institution on Slovene soil, the *Academia Operosorum*, was established, using as its coat of arms the castle of Ljubljana and a beehive, the latter depicted as being no less important than the castle. To this very day there are still bees flying high above the city. The members of the Academy, wishing to be as creative as bees, adopted for themselves the honourable title of *Apes academicae*, or 'academic bees'. In the nineteenth century bees were taken as an example by three cultural publications – in Ljubljana by the *Carniolian Bee (Kranjsko Cebelico)*, in Klagenfurt by the *Slovene Bee (Slovensko Bcelo)*, and in Celje by another *Slovene Bee*. Bees, beekeeping, honey and certainly that most ancient of drinks, Carniolian mead, were all described, in terms of highest praise, by the chronicler Johann Freihher von Valvasor in his work *The Honour of the Duchy of Carniola* in the year 1689. And, finally, Slovenia is the home of the renowned strain of bees known as *Apis mellifica carnica*.

To take up my story, I must picture myself sitting beneath a shady old tree on the scorched grass, where I had sat so many times before. There were a few chairs in the garden under the trees and two of them were occupied by two boxes tied to long poles. These boxes were full of bees which the keeper had just taken down from the trees. The bees were dizzy, for they had just completed the difficult duty of assuring the continuity of the race.

The time had come, they had decided, to fly off from the old home. Tired after a year of communal life, the living cloud had departed to find a branch where they could join their queen.

A murmuring came from the boxes which, at a glance, seemed to be quite still, but in reality they were continuously and restlessly quivering. The third chair was empty but prepared to receive a new family. This family was hanging like a heavy bunch of grapes just below the top of the biggest apple tree and Cene was trying to persuade them into the third box. He was trying to shake them off with one single, deft move so that most of the bees, with their queen, would fall into the box together and it would afterwards be merely a question of having to wait for the remainder to join the family.

We were silent. Words would have spoiled this solemn moment created by the restless murmurings of the bees in the box, the rhythmic droning from the hives, the playful dance of sunlight and shade in the tops of the apple trees and, perhaps, a reflection of all this in ourselves. Beside a tree trunk, in the shade of course, lay a bottle of original home-made schnapps and a couple of glasses so that anyone could help himself. The schnapps had a pleasant smell and was just strong enough to burn the lips, but each gulp refreshed the dry mouth and a little later warmed the whole body.

When Cene had collected the last of the swarm, when they had all settled and quietened, when the keeper had helped them into their new homes, he lit himself a cigarette. He puffed with great contentment and decided that the day's work was done. The talk began.

It was certainly not of war, which ever rages in one or other part of the world, neither was it of the ever-present economic problems which threaten us. No, we spoke of bees, and only of bees, for there was a peace in that village which also filled our own minds.

Someone remembered and mentioned propolis. He had read somewhere that it was widely used, or at least tried, and that it helped with many different illnesses. Much we heard and some, but not all, we believed.

Cene was quiet. He smiled at us, at the bees and at the last rays of the afternoon sun which were already slanting through the green treetops. He spoke only when really necessary. He listened to the story of the old beekeeper who supposedly ate the deadly green death-cap mushroom mixed up with some other mushrooms and did not die because he allowed himself plenty of brandy in which he had mixed propolis.

He thought a little longer, then added his own view on the wisdom of using propolis. 'It stands to reason that the stuff must have been beneficial, because everything the bees give us is good. Yet there has never been and never will be a simple cure for all diseases. We don't have doctors just for fun! They have to study for a long time to learn what to do for someone who has eaten the wrong mushrooms, or broken his leg. Go first to a doctor and then perhaps try tea or schnapps with propolis – they might be better!'

Calmly, with slow and heavy steps, he moved to the apiary and shortly returned with a very ordinary cardboard box in his hands. 'Look, isn't that beautiful?' He asked us, showing us what he had scraped up in the last year.

The tiny flakes sparkled in the last fading rays of the setting sun, transparent, of every different colour and shade, fragrant, clear as crystal – a supply of tiny flakes which every year the bees use to gum across the crevices in the honeycomb foundations in the hive. They are gathered carefully so that not the smallest speck goes astray.

'I still don't know what I'll do with it,' he said absently. 'Perhaps I really will soak it in alcohol, or maybe sell it. Certainly there's no hurry; it's so beautiful as it is, just to look at it from time to time.'

CHAPTER TWO

REDISCOVERY AND REJECTION

There are many ways for a man to become involved with bees, but perhaps the simplest and least unusual is to have had both a father and grandfather who were beekeepers – to have beekeeping in the family, so it is merely a matter of stepping out onto the well-worn path.

As for me, I became a beekeeper on account of a song, a song which the bees sing; on account of the quiet, ceaseless murmur in the tops of the flowering cherry and apple trees, as harmonious as countless soft strings; on account of the hidden murmurings in a calm sea of sweet-smelling buckwheat, the expectancy of the muffled roaring in the deep chamber. There was one bee, though, which hindered my progress by stinging my father, who was allergic to bees, on his bare toe, so that for ten minutes or more his tongue was numb.... Henceforth bees were forbidden in the house!

Rado Seifert came to bees by way of painting. He was a church painter, restoring paintings, refurbishing statues and painting murals. In his twenty-eighth year he met a farmer from Dolsko who was also a beekeeper and who asked him to restore a shrine and repaint the plaster statue of the Mother of God on it.

'If you do it well, after my death you will have two hives from my apiary,' he promised. When he died a few months later, his children respected this wish. So the way was paved; and within a year he had fourteen hives.

PROPOLIS, THE HEALER

Then, one day, Seifert's health was threatened – something strange began to happen to his left leg, his feet and toes. The skin became increasingly dark purple, finally almost black; his toes were ice-cold, completely without feeling, and on one a large, infected ulcer opened up and refused to heal. Every week he went to the doctor, who put ointment on the ulcer, jabbed his leg with needles and established that it really was without feeling. It was finally recommended, apparently as the only possibility, that half the leg be amputated straight away.

Seifert refused the operation and put on his boots. He would not give up so quickly. At home he covered his leg with honey, containing propolis, and bandaged it. After a few days, when he took off the bandages and cleaned his leg, he couldn't believe his eyes. The ulcer on his toe was gone, healed; his foot was warmer than before and no longer hurt him when he stood firmly on the floor. Once more he went to the doctor, and there was no further talk of amputation. He could not resist saying, as he walked out, 'If ever someone else comes with the same problem, try honey first – time enough for the scalpel later!'

As he had done before this mishap to his leg, Seifert went on visiting his bees, but now he saw them in a new light. The bees became a precious fount of health and each single hive became for him a drug factory, a well-stocked pharmacy. He knew a lot already but he was to make other discoveries. He wanted to delve deeper into the hive and its secrets.

THE FIRST EXPERIMENT

He built a special hive, with only one honeycomb and a glass cover, so that he could study the bees. Whenever he had time, he admired the activities within his glass-covered comb. He saw how the bees carried their load of pollen and plastered it down, how they filled the cells with sweet nectar gathered from countless flowers. He followed the journey of the queen bee from one cell to another among the workers, which thronged about her. All this he had already known and he could explain it all. Then he noticed that one bee placed an extremely small droplet of liquid on the frame of the comb. Another bee came and began to creep with the shining stuff into a fresh new cell which was waiting for an egg. It took about a minute to finish this task and the cell shone brightly, as if someone had lacquered it.

It had not been nectar which the first bee had brought in his pollen-basket, for honey does not shine and the bee would not coat the floor and walls of the cell with it. Rado Seifert was not a man to take a guess when he could just as easily test something, so he removed the glass and, with a piece of wood, rubbed off the remainder of the substance which the bee had brought in. It smelled good, though was not as sweet as honey on the tongue. What was it then that the bees had brought into the cell to make it a more pleasant home for the next generation?

He remembered the unknown substance later when, as happened every year, he cleaned the combs. With a knife he scraped from the wood and cell foundation a small heap of the substance which the bees had laid down and glued there. The resin had a pleasant smell, exactly like that of the tiny drop left in the glass-covered comb. When he tried it, it was again that slightly bittersweet taste in the mouth. This resin, he decided, must be propolis, about which he had read somewhere.

It did seem, he thought, that the bees must have a good reason for using the liquid as a sealing compound. So, when his wife burned her fingers with boiling oil and there was nothing suitable in the house to put on it, he had used some of the resinous liquid as an ointment. Soon his wife's fingers stopped hurting and in a few days there remained scarcely any visible trace of the burn.

The resin scraped from the frame, shingle and comb foundation of his apiary was therefore not, as was generally thought, and as the church painter himself had thought, a waste product of honey from which the bees made a lacquer. It did, in fact, possess remarkable healing properties, albeit unknown and untried.

Perhaps he should keep his secret to himself, for it seemed to him that if he told his story the best response he could hope for was indulgent laughter. (Indeed many beekeepers and doctors are still not convinced that propolis is a special medicine.) But he decided to go to the local doctor with his discovery.

He put two or three handsful of the pure substance into a bag and set off on his visit. He sat sipping coffee and talking about bees, the crops and honey before cautiously suggesting: 'Look, Max, I've brought you this to try. It's quite fresh, I scraped it off only a few days ago. I think you might find it worth trying as a medicine. You have enough patients in the hospital – you can easily find out which ones it will help.'

It was a big relief to have confided his thoughts to the

doctor. Quietly and patiently he waited for an answer.
Doctor Max Kern shook his head firmly.

CHAPTER THREE

THE FIRST CONVERT

'What are we going to do now, Barbara?' asked Uncle Max. The little girl, only four years old, was lying curled up in her father's armchair, almost asleep but moving restlessly, sometimes trembling violently. Anything that was said she could hear only from a distance, or perhaps not at all.

She lay there, feeling as if she was falling faster and faster into a horrible, black, bottomless pit. In the morning, when she had been wakened to go to kindergarten, she felt dizzy. 'She'll be sick again,' her father said, and he knew something about sickness because he was a dentist. Her mother and father decided that she must stay at home. Her throat hurt when she swallowed; even when her mother boiled her an egg she pushed the tray away. She wouldn't eat a bread roll either – nothing but water, tea, or milk, for she was terribly thirsty and hot. By midday she was no better, but she wanted more and more to drink because she was still thirsty.

Then a neighbour, Uncle Max, her father's doctor friend, came to visit her.

Now, if Uncle Max had been in the hospital, wearing his white coat and surrounded by lots of small bottles and other things, she would have been afraid; but here he was only an uncle, even if he did have a spoon in his hand and wanted her to show him her tongue. With a little persuasion and a few tears in her eyes, Barbara opened her mouth and said 'Aaaaah'. Uncle Max pressed the spoon on her tongue and looked so deeply into her mouth that he might easily have seen right down into her stomach. Then, shaking his head, he said, 'Yes, yes, just as I thought!'

'Bad tonsillitis again, isn't it?' her father sighed. 'That's the fourth time this year. When's it going to stop!'

It was true, Barbara had often had to stay in bed with tonsillitis. Before it had been a simple inflammation of the throat, without suppuration but, because of the frequency of the attacks, the infection began to suppurate. Almost always, her father would bring some tablets from his medicine chest and Barbara had to take them, even though they were bitter and difficult to swallow. Sometimes the doctor would come with an injection which he put deep under her skin.

'She's quite hot,' the doctor said. Her father had already taken her temperature. 'It's 39.7 degrees (103°F) he said, 'you'll have to give her something.'

A SWEET TREATMENT
Uncle Max stopped pondering, gave a hopeful, friendly glance at Barbara's feverish eyes, and asked, 'Now Barbara, what will you have? An injection or a sweet?'

Immediately she brightened. A smile appeared on her face, even if she hadn't understood why he was asking such a question. There is probably not one child on earth who would have to think twice before answering such a question. Barbara simply said that she would prefer a sweet.

'You'll have to give her something,' said her father again, 'You can't let her wait like this till tomorrow.'

'Of course we'll have to help Barbara,' said Uncle Max, smiling, 'You heard her. She probably knows best what will help her. She must be absolutely full of antibiotics. Let's try something different!'

Mother brought a lump of sugar from the kitchen and Uncle Max checked his pockets until he found a brown bottle. He put a few drops of pleasant-smelling liquid on the sugar and offered the now brown cube to Barbara, who took it cautiously and put it in her mouth. Nothing burned her, it tasted just like a real sweet, much better than bitter pills or painful injections.

While she slept the dentist and the doctor drank coffee and talked of many things. Two hours later they awakened the peacefully sleeping child and gave her another of Uncle Max's special sugar cubes. Her father took her temperature and couldn't believe his eyes: in only two hours it had fallen from 39.7 (103°F) to 37.6 degrees (99.7°F). All night the child slept quietly, woke naturally in the morning and, as usual, asked her mother to take her to kindergarten.

'Wait a moment, sweetheart,' her father smiled, 'we must see if you have a temperature.'

OVERNIGHT SUCCESS
But she hadn't. The thermometer showed no more than 37°C (98.4°F)! No high temperature. No more dizziness, no more pain, only an enormous appetite. She was so hungry that she ate everything her mother put in front of

her and even demanded more. Her mother and father exchanged happy glances; never before had she recovered so quickly.

However, they did not take her to the kindergarten, as she had wanted, but went instead to the health clinic for a check-up with an ear, nose and throat specialist.

'Why have you brought this child?' asked the surprised doctor. 'There's nothing the matter with her. The mucous membranes are nicely firm, no trace of infection in her tonsils. She's perfectly healthy.' Her mother had nothing to say, apart from thanking the doctor, and she left the clinic satisfied.

That evening she went to see her neighbour and reported: 'We were almost told off for going to the hospital for a check-up. Barbara is going back to kindergarten tomorrow.' Then she asked if Max could leave her some of the medicine, in case Barbara should have another attack of tonsillitis.

He gave her a medicine bottle and, to satisfy her curiosity, told her what it was. 'Actually nothing very special, just propolis dissolved in alcohol. It's something that comes from the beehives.'

Perhaps ten or more years passed by. Barbara was no longer little Barbara, no longer at kindergarten but in secondary school, and next year she would finish there too. Uncle Max was no longer 'Uncle' to her but 'Doctor'. Yet one thing had not changed – Max still believed in the powers of his sweets, and also in ointments, capsules and various other medicines containing his precious, natural healer, propolis.

DOCTOR'S DILEMMA

Dr Max Kern had been presented with something of a dilemma following his emphatic refusal to experiment with the sample of propolis that Rado Seifert had brought to him a decade ago. As an orthodox doctor he had up to then been practising medicine the way he had learned it at university, as he saw it practised in hospitals, as described in medical text books and journals; in short, as medical science had ordered it. Neither at the university, nor in the better-known medical journals had there ever been mention of propolis, and even if he believed it might be of some use, he could never dare to try it on his patients. Such things were forbidden and, in any case, his sense of responsibility was against it – patients are not guinea pigs to be experimented on! But, by chance, a subsequent event had caused him to look again at this remarkable substance which he had firstly waved aside.

Rado Seifert was a stubborn man, and he was very insistent about his sample of dark brown scrapings from the hives. The propolis was sticky and wax-like and to the doctor its only advantage had seemed to be its pleasant smell. Rado had a strong conviction that it would prove to be a good medicine, and it is just as well that he pressed his case, for otherwise Dr Kern would probably still be treating small Barbaras with tonsillitis with bitter-tasting tablets or injections, instead of offering them pleasant-smelling sugar cubes.

'How are we going to purify this stuff?' Rado had asked, and they both had suggested simultaneously, 'Why not try alcohol?'

Rado did not have alcohol from the pharmacy in mind, however. He had been thinking of home-made brandy, which he himself made from fruit, from the half-ripe apples which fell off the trees, the pears which were

21

already bad when picked, all mixed with over-ripe plums shaken from the trees. If nothing else, he had thought it would be interesting to offer his neighbours a brandy with not only the characteristic taste and smell of the fruit but also the pleasant and unusual aroma of various forest resins. But the doctor had insisted on having his way – if it was ever to be tried at all, it would have to be seriously undertaken, and in the end they dissolved the 'rubbish' in pure alcohol.

'You will try it in the hospital, won't you?' Rado had urged, to which the doctor had replied, 'Oh no I won't!'

'But it won't harm anyone,' Rado had protested, trying to change the doctor's mind.

'Maybe that's true. Perhaps it won't do any harm, but I'm not going to try it!'

FATE TAKES A HAND

And probably it would never have been tried, the bottle of brown fluid would have remained on the store-room shelf until finally someone cleaning the store threw it out, if one day Doctor Kern had not decided to trim the hedge. He had to cut the hedge by hand, and as he was working away with the secateurs he suddenly felt a stab of pain in one of his fingertips, a sharp excruciating pain. Then blood started to run.

His hand opened and the secateurs fell to the ground. Cursing under his breath, he went to the tap, turned it on and put his bleeding hand under the water to wash off the dirt. Only then could he see that he really had more than just a bad cut on his fingertip; in fact, his fingertip was missing. Heaven alone knew where it had fallen. Searching with his good hand among the grass and hedge clippings he failed to find it. He stopped searching, picked up the secateurs and smiled wryly to himself, for there on the blade of the cutters, among bits of leaf and all the debris imaginable, was the piece of his finger.

He washed the amputated fingertip in water and pressed it back in place, wondering what he could put on to help it heal. Then he remembered the bottle with the solution of resin in it. Perhaps, he thought, it was true what Rado had said. What if propolis *did* work? If he couldn't try it on others, he could at least try it on himself. There was no law against that and no medical ethics to worry about either.

He brought the bottle from the store-room. He had no time to filter the liquid, so he poured some of it over his finger and again felt stinging pain. Not for long, though, for the pain soon stopped. He bandaged his finger and poured the propolis over the bandage many times.

As he started, so he intended to continue. He didn't take any other medicine as he otherwise would have. The experiment would be reliable only if he was consistent, so he would have to risk infection in order to test the effectiveness of the propolis.

When his fingertip became an angry, dark purple colour, Doctor Kern began to think that the lotion would not be successful and that he would give the bottle back to Rado to do whatever he wished with it. But on the third day, and even more so by the fourth day, the colour of his finger was noticeably paler. By the end of the week he no longer doubted that his fingertip would live! The finger gradually returned to normal, as it had been before the accident. His test, the first experiment, was completely successful.

A CONVERT TO PROPOLIS

When he finally removed the bandages altogether he did not return the bottle to Rado, as he had previously intended, but carefully stored it, no longer in the pantry among the preserved fruit, but in his medicine chest. Propolis had not yet, of course, achieved any acclaim but it had taken the first step on the long and difficult road to recognition. Even with Dr Kern, it was only half-recognition, which is understandable. Since a finger is only a finger and his wound had been a relatively minor one, he felt that with something more serious, it would be far safer to stay on the beaten track of medical science and knowledge.

A TEST ON TONSILLITIS

When propolis was next put to the test it concerned not a mere finger, but Annette, the Doctor's only daughter. When she was healthy, she was a lively, if sensitive child. However, sad to say, she often had to stay in bed when her friends were playing in the park or throwing snowballs in the winter. She suffered attack after attack of tonsillitis, up to ten times a year, really too much for a small girl.

Her father had decided that there was probably no other remedy than to have the tonsils removed, but always he postponed taking the final step, always something unexpected occurred. The attacks of tonsillitis continued month after month, right up to the week when the family were due to go on holiday. The night before their departure, Annette was again in bed with a temperature of 39°C (102°F).

As before, antibiotics should have helped and she was given a bigger dose than usual. The family postponed the holiday, though, as Annette's fever was more persistent than usual. By the third morning her temperature had climbed higher, and her anxious mother reminded her husband of the medicine he and Rado Seifert had prepared.

'What? Propolis?' Dr Kern was surprised. 'Why should we use that? I know best what will cure her.'

'Remember what it did for your finger,' she prompted, but he was unconvinced.

'A finger is only a finger, and that was an injury. I just had to put the propolis on the outside to cure it. This illness is caused by microbes and for that we fortunately have antibiotics.'

The doctor decided to increase the dose of antibiotics for Annette, but when her husband went out Mrs Kern took matters into her own hands. She soaked a sugar cube in propolis until it was yellowish-brown and gave it to Annette. An hour or so later she repeated this procedure and waited for results. At lunchtime, when her husband came home from the hospital to eat, she told him that she had given some of Rado's medicine to Annette.

'So you think you know best?' he said angrily, 'Alright, you treat her, if you think you know more about medicine than I do. But don't ask me any more what should be done for Annette!'

Of course he didn't really mean what he said, but was afraid to show his interest in the unusual remedy. He strained to observe his daughter out of the corner of his eye but refused to examine her closely. He paced up and down the flat, muttering to himself about antibiotics and propolis in an effort to impress his wife. Before he returned to the hospital he went quickly to the bedside and put his hand on the child's forehead, which was enough to make a quick diagnosis. Certainly she was no worse, although she had had no more antibiotics since morning.

Two days later the family left the city on their holiday.

As they drove down to the coast, Dr Kern remarked to his wife, 'You know, the antibiotics really did help her. I gave her more than usual and it took longer, but she got much better when they finally started to work.' His wife was not concerned with the honour of the medical profession, only with her daughter's health, so she made no comment.

An appointment had already been made for Annette to go into hospital to have her tonsils removed, but they kept postponing the date because she had no further attacks of tonsillitis.

That autumn a friend of Annette's came to stay, who had trouble with her throat in spite of the fact that her tonsils had been removed. Doctor Max was at first surprised that her throat was sore, because her tonsils had gone, but then he discovered that the operation had not been entirely successful. A small part of the tonsils still remained, swollen and infected.

'You know what? We'll try the same cure we used for Annette in the summer. Antibiotics didn't help much that time and propolis did. For a while we'll settle for the sugar cubes; if that doesn't work there'll be time for other medicines later!'

There was no need for anything else.

His wife could hardly stop herself from laughing aloud. When Annette had been ill it had been quite a different story!

Since then Doctor Max has many, many times asked his young patients casually, 'So, what will you have now? An injection or a sweet?'

CHAPTER FOUR

NEW HORIZONS FOR PROPOLIS

The excellent results of using propolis on the amputated finger, the throat infection, other types of inflammatory diseases and the everyday scratches and injuries to children's knees, hands or elbows all combined to demonstrate to Dr Max Kern that propolis was powerfully effective against inflammation, was also successful against bacteria and, used directly against inflammation or infection, it was as effective – and frequently more effective than – pharmaceutical antibiotics. He confirmed the astonishingly rapid action of propolis, that it either relieved or entirely prevented pain and, of particular importance, that it seemed to him that neither children nor adults experienced any difficulties in taking it.

The human organism was, therefore, not allergic to propolis, making it very different from other antibiotics which frequently give rise to various, sometimes very unpleasant, reactions in sensitive people.

SKIN TROUBLES
Then it happened that his fourteen-year-old daughter, as often happens with girls of that age, began to be daily

harrassed by a great anxiety. No, it was not her health which was at stake, but her beauty. She developed the most unpleasant spots on her face, and later on her back. For young people entering maturity this is the most distressing of all problems; indeed, they can scarcely conceive of anything worse. At exactly the time when they most want to be beautiful and attractive to others, their soft, smooth, clear skin vanishes and becomes covered with blemishes, so that all they want to do is hide away in a dark place. Parents, doctors, and everyone else advise fresh water, clean air, walks, fruit and vegetables, and all of them absolutely forbid these quite distraught teenagers to squeeze the inflamed spots, lest they become infected.

Sufferers will turn to any remedy at this time – creams, lotions, ointments, anything. Annette decided that she would try something different, something her father always kept in a dark brown bottle in the medicine cupboard.

One evening she soaked a pad of cotton wool with the liquid and carefully smeared it on the spots on her face. It gave her skin an unusual colour, not its normal rosy pink, but a patchy yellow, darker where she had dabbed it more than once with the damp pad. She wondered if it would wash off and worried a little about what her father would say if he noticed that quite a lot of his lotion had been used. But at fourteen no risk is too great to acquire a beautiful skin.

In the morning she got out of bed earlier than normal and of her own accord, though usually her mother had to call her two or three times and then pull the blankets off before she would get up. She went first to the mirror and looked at herself; she looked again and considered. Certainly her face was yellow but the infected pimples had entirely gone, leaving behind small reddish traces, and they were dry. There was enough propolis in her father's bottle to use again that night – she could wash her face and be beautiful.

Her father indeed noticed that the bottle was nearly empty and he was afraid that someone had been drinking the solution. Then he noticed that the ugly rash on Annette's face had dried up and that her skin was clear. He didn't know whether to be angry on account of the small empty bottle or happy on account of his daughter's skin. And there was a third reaction, namely his enthusiasm at having found yet another use for propolis. Perhaps Rado or some other beekeeper would allow him to scrape some more of the substance from the hives.

'You must help me. We need more propolis! For all the tonsillitis, scratched knees and still more for your skin!' he explained to Annette. For he surely knew that acne is not an illness which may be cured once and for all, but one which will occur again and again, as long as there are growing teenagers.

After they had been to a beekeeper and scraped the resin from his hives, Dr Kern began to wonder how else he could use the miraculous cure. Perhaps other complaints would respond to treatment with propolis.

A DENTAL DISASTER
Then, once again, fate stepped into his life. Well, not exactly fate, but a 68-year-old neighbour, a pensioner from across the street. Age, always a merciless enemy of teeth, was partly to blame, but the old lady herself was also wrong. It is true that hardly anyone likes to go to the dentist, but this old lady was especially afraid. She did not expect to live much longer, being already elderly, and thought that as long as she did live she would be able to

use her well-worn teeth. She did not use them any more for anything hard, having given up eating meat or biting apples, and even the worst teeth were good enough for eating bread dipped in milky coffee.

It became apparent, however, that her calculations were not very accurate and that the old lady had far more life left in her body than power in her teeth. They hurt, more so every day, so that she could no longer say exactly where and what hurt. With a heavy heart she decided to go to the dentist to ask him to do the best he could.

'Oh dear, you should have come sooner,' he scolded her in a gentle tone, 'About twenty years ago, in fact. But it's no good crying over spilt milk; we'll take them all out and then make you such a fine set of false ones that you'll be able to crack walnuts again!'

She did not protest, whatever he did, not even when he explained that he would take out simultaneously and without an injection, five and a half decayed old roots. The X-ray had shown that these were infected and for this reason he strongly advised against an anaesthetic.

She put up with everything that was necessary, though the pain really was very severe. She even thought that it would have been considerably easier after all if she had been to the dentist twenty, or perhaps even thirty, years earlier. But what must be must be! When she left, swallowing blood clots which she found in her mouth, she consoled herself that the worst was over.

It wasn't! An hour later the pain in her lacerated lower jaw was worse; in the beginning she seemed to feel a swelling with her tongue and slowly the swelling grew worse and the pain even sharper, almost unbearable. She wanted to go back to the dentist but it was already too late – the surgery hours were over and the clinic closed. What could she do? Who would help her? It was too long to wait till tomorrow. Of course! She would go across the road to Dr Kern. He was a good man and he would have already left the hospital and be at home. Certainly he was not a dentist, but he was a doctor and every doctor must have on hand something good, maybe even better than the things sold in the pharmacy.

The doctor in her street had a medicine that was not available from any chemist's shop. He had a full bottle of propolis! She dabbed the few drops of the unknown liquid on her lacerated, swollen, painful gums, as the doctor had advised, and waited.

It didn't hurt anymore! The pain which had seemed unbearable before had disappeared without trace.

Next morning she made herself some tea, as the doctor had suggested. She had already soaked some bread in warm milk but, even though it was the soft part of the loaf with no crust, she could scarcely bring herself to try it. But later she put the crust into the milk and waited a little for it to soften; then she ate it all, just as if her jaws were undamaged and had teeth in them.

Maybe four or five times a day she put the liquid propolis on her gums. Her lower jaw remained uninfected and healed quickly, returning to normal size. Four days later she went fearlessly back to the dentist for a check-up.

The dentist was surprised to see her unworried and in good spirits, but when he looked in her mouth he was even more amazed. The lacerations where he had extracted the roots of her long-neglected teeth were scarcely noticeable. He could not understand it and wanted to know what she had done. She told him how painful it had been and what sort of medicine she had been given. Anything more than that she couldn't explain.

CURE FOR AN ULCER

A day or two later propolis was also able to help a twelve-year-old and his stomach. He was an attractive and lively child, until he started to complain of pains in his tummy after meals. In the beginning his parents didn't worry very much, even though his father was a doctor and a child specialist at that.

'He's been eating too much,' the father decided. He never imagined that it could be anything serious. However, when the boy became unusually subdued and his marks at school dropped, when he spent too much of his time at home lying on the couch after meals and leaving the table during meals, his father realized that something *was* wrong. The boy, Josht, said that he felt bloated and had burning pains in his stomach. He was taken to the gastro-enterological clinic for a thorough examination. The clinical findings and the X-rays revealed the same thing: an ulcer of the small intestine!

The clinic suggested some drugs to his father and these were obtained. Josht took them readily and felt better; the distension of his stomach went away and the pain ceased. But, when he stopped taking the medicine, within a day everything was just as it had been before. He was ill again, apathetic, the despair of his parents. And this process repeated itself until one day, in conversation with a colleague from another clinic, the father began to talk of his son's difficulties.

His colleague Dr Kern said, thinking aloud, 'Who knows, maybe propolis would help him; it certainly wouldn't do any harm!'

A little louder he explained: 'If you like we could try him with propolis. It's not a medicine, at least not officially, and you won't get it at a pharmacy; but it's helped a lot of people. I don't know what would happen with a stomach ulcer.'

Instead of medicine, Josht now took ten to fifteen drops of propolis on a sugar cube, three times a day. It was as effective as the medicine he had previously taken and for more than a week there was no repetition of his stomach trouble. For some weeks they treated the boy with a capsule of propolis three times a day, a quarter of an hour before meals. Then he ceased to have any trouble, was eating as before and doing well at school.

His father noticed something else interesting. For some years the boy had had quite a lot of nasal trouble, and a specialist had diagnosed vasomotor rhinitis, but no drugs were prescribed to help his breathing. After he had been taking propolis his breathing was not so heavy, he began breathing through his nose more normally and easily, and the nasality of his speech disappeared. Had propolis contributed to his vastly improved condition? Perhaps the release of etheric substances in the oral cavity acted upon the nasal membranes in such a way as to clear infection of the nose, decrease nasal secretions, finally opening the nasal passages enough to allow easy breathing.

For proof of this we will have to wait, as we must also wait for a number of other explanations about how propolis functions and how to assure favourable results from its hidden powers of healing.

CHAPTER FIVE

A SICK CHILD

Although buckwheat is called *ajda* and is eaten as a cereal in Slovene, it is in fact not a cereal at all, even if it does give us porridge and flour for bread. Its home is in the cold Himalayan mountains and along the shores of Lakes Amur and Bajkal but, surprisingly, it is not a strong, tenacious plant, but delicate and sensitive to frosts. It is a source of nourishment for both man and bee, offering to the latter its pink and white flowers as the last autumnal pasture.

Then there is another Ajda, not a cereal either. Unlike our natural *ajda* (*Phagopyrum esculentum*), this is not at all delicate and sensitive and is far more like the other wild and stubborn plants of the Himalayas. She is, in fact, a lively nine-year-old girl and my own daughter.

Nevertheless, despite her hardy constitution, the doctor had often told Ajda not to go to school but to stay at home. Of course it was always others who were to blame, as in the instance of her schoolfriend who caught scarlet fever, putting her neighbours in quarantine lest they too catch it. Many girls from the class caught the

34

disease, but Ajda ran happily round the garden until the incubation period was over. Those days were wonderful for her, full of freedom and with plenty of her mother's attention. We all watched her, waiting for the tell-tale headache or temperature, the first signs of the red rash; but nothing happened, except that she scratched her leg badly and nearly broke every bone in her body when a tree branch broke, sending her plummeting to the ground like a sack.

But she was no exception to the rule and of course could be taken by surprise by illness, even when there were no illnesses at school.

CHILDHOOD ILLNESS

The first sign that something was wrong this time was that she did not eat her breakfast, said she just could not eat because her mouth was sore. She couldn't tell us exactly what was wrong. Although her throat seemed all right, her gums were perhaps a little too red.

Next day Ajda had a high temperature, the thermometer showing 40 degrees (104°F.). Inside her lips and particularly on her gums were small red pustules. Her gums were a pronounced red, smarted and were covered by what looked like a fine cobweb of lacerated and purulent membranes. When she ate some bread there were traces of blood everywhere.

She tossed restlessly in her bed, trying unsuccessfully to sleep. One tablet, and another, from our household pharmacy helped to ease her fever but the inflammation of her gums increased and the pain grew worse. Even this unyielding and stubborn little girl could no longer keep back the tears which gathered silently in her eyes.

A doctor came and, shaking her head, wrote a prescription. Tablets for the temperature, gentian violet as an embrocation, an antibiotic and quite a large dose of a vitamin B-complex tablet to be taken with the antibiotic, and in four days time another medical examination. Her mother bought everything the doctor had prescribed and I myself was to give her the tablets and paint her gums.

I gathered up all my courage, put on my spectacles and took all the medicines, a glass of water, a spoon and some sterilized wadding, to Ajda's bedside. I could see clearly that she was afraid, however impatiently she was awaiting the help of the medicines. I tried not to look inside her wide eyes because her every look hurt me also. I thought how easy it would be if I were simply a doctor at work, but even a doctor would feel upset at having to treat his own child.

I was quite clumsy, making my preparations impossibly slowly. Then I unexpectedly remembered discussing propolis and I thought over all that had been said. Yes, propolis was said to have an anti-inflammatory effect. If Ajda's disease had been caused by a representative of the strange world of microbes, propolis would once again be the most suitable remedy. If the tiny, scarcely visible sores on her gums were to be healed, nothing would work more rapidly than propolis. Ajda said that everything was painful and perhaps propolis would ease the pain.

'Wait, Ajda, if you don't mind we'll try another way,' I told her. 'The medicines Mamma has bought are probably very good but we'll keep them for some other time. Let's say until tomorrow or the day after, should my medicine not work. You agree?'

Why wouldn't she when that meant that I would take away the nasty bottle of purple liquid and all the other paraphernalia? My wife objected and thought that the child should take the medicines which she needed and

36

which were real medicines. The doctor should know what was right and I should not interfere in her affairs. But she could not alter anything, since Ajda and I had already come to an agreement.

First I put quite a few drops of propolis solution into half a glass of water. Ajda watched carefully how the propolis dissolved into the water, turning it milky white. Wanting her to trust me, I took a gulp first myself and said how tasty it was. Then Ajda drank a few drops and discovered that it did not burn at all, was not bitter and was, on the whole, quite pleasant, because it cooled her sore lips and gums. She washed out her mouth diligently for some ten minutes, holding fresh solution in her mouth as long as she could then spitting it out, resting a moment and then taking another gulp.

'You can see for yourself now that propolis isn't bad,' I said, preparing her for the following, less pleasant, treatment. 'Of course it's not the propolis but the alcohol which is going to hurt a little. If you grit your teeth you'll be able to stand it better, but it will all be over quickly,' I promised her, trying to be helpful.

She clenched her teeth and pulled back her open lips so that I could quickly paint all the inflammation. I knew the alcohol stung badly for a few moments and that even the most gentle touch of the wadding on the sore places must have hurt her a lot. But she stood it as long as she could then started to cry, spitting a pink salivary liquid into a basin.

I stroked her hair, talking comfortingly to her. I told her it was all over, that it had to hurt a little, and that there must be a few drops of blood in her saliva if her gums were all lacerated. For this reason everything would be better later, the pain would go, she would be able to get up and also be able to eat.

She settled down and promised me that next time she would grit her teeth and not cry. Of course, it would have been easier if she only had to wash her mouth out with the milky-white fluid, but that might be no use.

For another quarter of an hour I had to tell her all about the strange medicine which the bees give us and also about the bees themselves. Then she pulled at my hand and laughed: 'Daddy, your medicine worked! It doesn't hurt any more! Have a look, maybe I'm better!'

I tried to convince her that not even propolis could work so quickly. But the pain had really gone and she ate without any problems.

When her temperature was normal she got up, but we continued our treatment three or four times a day in the bathroom. It hurt every time and the tears always came involuntarily to her eyes, yet afterwards, when she looked in the mirror, she could see that the rash was diminishing, that there was less and less of the ugly cobweb on her gums, and that the flesh was no longer such a blood red colour.

SURPRISE DIAGNOSIS

After the fourth day we went to see the doctor who had visited Ajda on the second day of her illness.

'Well my dear, is it still bad?' she asked her, and Ajda answered by nodding her head impishly. 'I'm afraid it will last; it doesn't go away so quickly,' the doctor informed her. Then, looking in her mouth, 'It's incredible,' she marvelled, 'it's nearly cleared up, though it usually takes quite a lot longer. It's healing very nicely.'

Then her expression changed from surprise to doubt. She stopped looking with satisfaction at Ajda and looked straight into my eyes. 'Listen, gentian violet always leaves traces behind, but I don't see any dye in her mouth. Did you paint it on as I advised? Did you buy the medicine?'

I was a little embarrassed and spoke quietly: 'Of course we bought the medicine. I've got the bottle at home in the cupboard but it's still full. You see, Ajda got better without it.'

'What about the vitamin B? Surely you gave her the antibiotic as I prescribed. If you had put that in the cupboard instead of giving it to the child, Ajda's condition would be much worse now than four days ago.'

It would have been better if we had peacefully gone home at that moment. The doctor would have been a little angry but Ajda and I could have laughed a little together. But I had to tell her everything about propolis, because it was true.

'The vitamin B is also in the cupboard. Ajda took two or three tablets for the fever but otherwise it was propolis which really worked. I bathed her mouth with it and sprayed her gums with it. It burned a little, but it helped.'

For a moment there was silence, as if she hadn't understood me. The doctor put her hand to her spectacles, moved them a little, scratched her eyebrow with one finger and finally removed her spectacles altogether. She looked at me strangely and distrustfully.

'What did you say? Propolis? I've never heard of that preparation. Did you get it from the United States, or perhaps from Russia? We get too little information about their new drugs.'

'No, just from a beehive,' I assured her, 'Yes, really, from a beehive, from bees, our own at home.'

Then we talked for a long time, not about Ajda and her illness, but about propolis. She was interested in everything about it, although she was not convinced that all I told her was true. Perhaps our conversation could have been longer and more thorough but we had to stop as there were more people in the waiting room who had come for help.

'Well, come again soon if Ajda isn't all right,' she ordered and I promised her a bottle of propolis solution.

As it happened I didn't have to go to the clinic with Ajda again. For a day or two longer I painted her gums and washed out her mouth. Then everything was just as it had been before the disease.

But perhaps not. For in our family I was now no longer the only member who had a secret prescription for a medicine written under the code name 'propolis'.

MORE CONVERTS

Disciple number one of propolis is Ajda. She always takes care that there is a good supply of propolis in the cupboard and when she goes off to the holiday camp at the seaside in summer she takes a bottle with her – in case she steps on a sea-urchin, if any of her friends scratch their legs, if she has a sore throat and so on.

Her four-year-old brother Lan is no less convinced about propolis, though he prefers his propolis with honey, as in Melbrosin propolis or Apikompleks. If it seems that he may conceivably develop a sore throat, he begs, 'Daddy give me some propolis, please!' And he climbs up to take it from the cupboard himself. Well, the honey is sweet and the propolis is beneficial, so while his father treats little Lan this way at home he doesn't need to see a doctor.

And there is also a bottle of propolis solution in the cupboard where my wife keeps all her creams and lotions and lacquers and all her other aids to feminine beauty.

In our house nobody looks at me strangely or angrily if I suggest taking propolis, as happened when Ajda was ill. Quite the contrary, our troubles with propolis begin very differently. For instance: 'Daddy, a midge has fallen in my eye, give me some propolis.'

'Daddy, Jan threw a stone and it hit me on the leg and it hurts. Will you put some propolis on it please?'

'A dog has bitten my teddy-bear, can I give him a sugar cube with propolis?'

Then I have to show him that propolis is not a universal cure-all, that it does not promote eternal youth or heal broken bones and, in particular, that it will not help the white cloth teddy-bear which has not been bitten by a dog!

CHAPTER SIX

ACHIEVING MEDICAL RECOGNITION

The first medical success with propolis was in a gynaecological clinic in the Institute of Radiology at Sarajevo, where Dr Max Kern was assisted by Dr Izet Osmanagic and his colleagues.

They decided to use natural bee products on female patients who they were treating, either operatively or by radiation, for various malignant tumours of the womb, breast and ovaries. Despite the most stringent protective measures, the inevitable side-effects were occurring from these treatments, caused both by the radiation itself and also by poisoning from decaying matter from the radiated tissue. Of all organs, the liver was most affected; the blood cell count was lowered, digestive disturbances occurred, and so on – all of which could be detected by laboratory analysis. Many of the difficulties, such as tiredness, dizziness, head-ache, excitability, sleeplessness, digestive disturbances, and other unpleasant symptoms were obvious to the patients themselves, who sometimes became so exhausted that the doctor had to abandon the therapy.

For the first test 90 female patients were divided into three groups, the first receiving Florapoll capsules, a mixture of pollen and royal jelly, the second a well prepared placebo, and the third the classical treatment as before.

The second time they divided 44 patients into two groups. The first group received Melbrosin super, honey containing pollen and royal jelly, and the second, as before, a placebo. The results exceeded all expectations.

Among patients receiving the bee products symptoms either disappeared or were greatly alleviated; with other patients, however, the difficulties remained. Liver damage was absent among the first group and the lowering of the blood cell count was considerably less than with the other patients.

PROPOLIS AND RADIATION

Testing at the Institute of Oncology in Ljubljana also led to the investigation of bee products. In this case propolis in a honey preparation was used. A total of 37 patients receiving radiation treatment for malignant tumours of the oral cavity, tongue, and throat were chosen. An initial dosage of 4,000 rads was given and a few weeks later a stronger dosage of 6,800 rads was administered.

Such treatment is usually followed by an infection of the mucous membranes called *radium mucositis*, occurring after the sixth or seventh dose of radiation. Even small injuries to the mucous membrane are unbearably painful and a white or yellowish film of albumin forms. Because of the pain caused by swallowing, patients prefer to remain hungry, causing a weakening of the body's defence mechanisms and loss of weight. The blood cell count during radiation treatment drops by as much as 15 to 20 per cent.

Test patients received a teaspoonful of the honey preparation three times daily. The dose was kept in the mouth as long as possible, allowing it to dissolve in the saliva and move about the oral cavity and down the throat, coating the mucous membranes and permitting propolis to carry out its work.

Which of the ingredients of propolis was effective it is impossible to say, and the precise mechanism of the cure is also difficult to explain. Is perhaps the thin film which forms over areas which have had contact with propolis the most important thing? Does propolis merely protect against damage, or does it heal damage already caused? How is propolis effective against pain? Such questions are innumerable and, alas, the answers are few.

But surely the most important thing for a doctor, and even more so for the patient, is the result obtained from the use of a medicament. In the case of radium mucositis the effectiveness of propolis was proved beyond all doubt.

During the treatment with propolis, symptoms of illness were either completely absent or present only in mild forms. The critical stage of treatment, the sixth and seventh dosage of radiation, having been passed, the expected adverse changes remained almost unnoticeable but the treatment was as effective as usual. Even where heavy damage had occurred before the use of propolis the condition of the patient improved. In one case radiation treatment of a benign tumour of the tongue had resulted in serious inflammation, reddening of mucous membranes, burning, and intense pain for the patient. Treatment with propolis resulted in complete relief from pain, the burning ceased and the patient was able to eat normally.

Patients who passed through the critical phase of

radiation treatment without the usual difficulties – radium mucositis, loss of weight, weakness, disturbance of the blood cells – provide a convincing enough answer to the question of whether or not there is an effective substance for the treatment of the, until now inevitable, side-effects of radiation treatment. The bee had lent a helping hand to the rays, offering assistance to destroy what must be destroyed and easing the pain in that which must live.

Also in the gynaecological clinic in Sarajevo, a doctor was treating cervical damage with liquid propolis. Although the causes of such damage are various, the results are always the same – small sores which often grow to some centimetres in diameter with vigorous infection of the membranes, creating ideal conditions for the growth of cancer. The doctor reported that as many as forty patients, the youngest being twenty and the oldest forty-three years old, were cured after fifteen days of treatment. Mucous secretions became normal, infection disappeared and the troublesome sores healed overnight.

In short, every day propolis overcame some new challenge in the world of medicine.

CHAPTER SEVEN

PROPOLIS AND ULCERS

Everyone wore a white uniform, permanent staff and guests alike, although this was not a hospital and they all thought that it would have been better had they been dressed in fur coats as well. It was high summer outside but in the warehouse it was wintery. The factory had to be kept cool during processing of the honey, propolis and other bee products.

The visitors were shown the flower pollen, carefully wrapped in transparent bags. First they looked at the typical pollen which is collected by the bees from flowers, then at the processed, transformed variety Then they stopped at the stocks of propolis, collected from various sources and prepared for processing. After they had moved on from the refrigerated room they began a discussion about developments in research with propolis – how much chemists and microbiologists already knew and what doctors had discovered in their clinics.

'Well, propolis has been quite successful in curing duodenal and gastric ulcers,' the head of the laboratory put in. 'Dr Feiks from Klosterneuburg in Austria has done a large number of tests using samples of our product!'

'For ulcers we use a solution of propolis in water or milk,' explained a specialist adviser and doctor. He had some glasses ready and poured two fingers of water into each, then added a few drops of propolis solution. He mixed each one, producing a milky-coloured liquid which he offered to his guests. Slowly raising his glass he laughed, 'Friends, unfortunately this is not champagne but, anyway, cheers!'

The others also laughed and drank. Certainly there were better things to drink but, all in all, propolis was not without flavour. There were many jokes and much conjecturing about the outcome of their first experience of the unusual substance. But the minister who was there did not joke or make guesses, nor did he laugh with the rest; staring at the liquid, he drank it all in small sips, as if it was a precious medicine.

'Could I have some more of that sample?' he asked jokingly as he was leaving, but when he was given some his eyes lit up with new hope.

'Next week he has to go into hospital,' one of the guests whispered, nodding his head in the direction of the minister. 'He's got a duodenal ulcer which must be operated on a second time.'

The first operation had not helped for very long and soon the pain and bleeding had returned. The minister already had a second appointment, a bed was waiting for him in the hospital, and his name was already written down on the operating schedule. They told me, though that soon after he had got back to his office he had again tried some propolis, that he had taken it three times a day as the doctor had advised him. Perhaps he had recovered, they said, and I heard nothing more of the minister's illness.

THE MINISTER'S STORY

But I now know that he did not go to hospital as he should have done. The bed which was waiting for him had received a different patient and they postponed the operating schedule for the following week. They didn't operate on the minister that next week, nor the week after. More than a year passed since the discussion about propolis and the operation on his duodenum was still being postponed. Who knows till when – maybe for ever. Since the minister is still a young man, not even forty yet, it may be for quite a long time!

At about the same time they should have operated on a fifty-year-old man, a mechanic in a factory, who had a gastric ulcer. He had been suffering for quite a long time and the pain was increasing, so, as he was told, he first tried a change of diet. It seemed to him that he was forbidden nearly everything, but what the doctors did allow him, he rejected of his own accord. He lost weight all the more rapidly and the pain increased to a point where he was in despair. Then they told him that an operation would help and he agreed without giving it a second thought. A date was set but the man unexpectedly began to consider the matter and let them know that he would not come for the operation just yet.

What happened then?

Nothing very unusual: he just met a doctor who mentioned propolis and gave him a capsule containing a mixture of propolis and royal jelly. He tried it, at first only so that the doctor would not be angry with him, but after the first day the pain diminished. During the following days he was able to forget the troubles which had been torturing him for many years. He didn't have to worry about food any more; he ate everything, whatever the doctors had forbidden as well as what they had permitted

48

him. Before long they started teasing him at home – about the danger of his clothes becoming so small that he would have to buy new ones!

MODERN ILLS
All over the world there are millions of patients who are the victims of ulcers. These ulcers are a reflection of one of the most widespread diseases of our time. To attain the unattainable we are forever over-reaching the strength of our blood vessels, nerves and muscles. We also eat that which we should not, we breathe in poisons instead of air, we use our legs to drive a car instead of for walking. It is terrible that doctors meet young people of fourteen or fifteen who come to them with ulcers and ask for an operation.

If an ulcer is not a serious threat to life a doctor will not operate because he knows full well that within a few years it may have serious consequences – a continual diminishing of acidity or the sudden discovery of a cancerous growth! So a doctor will first recommend a diet which may inhibit pain, or a mild medication; he will hope that the body will join the fight and rid itself of the disease.

ULCER TREATMENT
Dr Franz Klemens Feiks is also trying out a new remedy for ulcers, in a hospital in the small picturesque Austrian town of Klosterneuberg. Dr Feiks is not only a doctor but a beekeeper and, above all, a man who believes that nature has provided man with many treasures for maintaining health.

Because he discovered from day to day how little patients with either gastric or duodenal ulcers were helped by the most marvellous drugs from pharmacies and factories, he decided to begin looking for help from the old and humble sources which have long been of benefit to mankind.

'What, propolis, is that a medicine?' they asked him in the beginning and he explained in his own way.

'Maybe propolis is a medicine, maybe it's not. I don't know and others don't know either. But why should we think of a medicine when we should be thinking of maintaining health? Why doesn't anyone ask me if the sun is a medicine? Why not ask if clear, fresh water or a breath of forest air is medicine? Or a shirt, sweat-stained from a mountain climb, a bite of a sunny apple, or a glass of milk? We must not ask or surmise too much; first we must live like people, then we will be healthy always!'

So he made no guesses as to what propolis really was; it was enough for him to know that it helped people in need, that it healed cuts and that it might also heal ulcers.

Dr Feiks therefore decided to use propolis to treat gastric and duodenal ulcers and chose exactly three hundred people for his experiment. Among them were six who were not yet twenty years old. Approximately a hundred had been afflicted for less than three years, the same number for three to ten years and a hundred more had been receiving treatment for more than a decade.

To avoid taking risks Dr Feiks decided that in the beginning he would give his patients the conventional diet and medication as well as propolis. To approximately half the patients he administered propolis three times a day before meals, always a water emulsion of propolis and alcohol in solution. Later, when he was certain of the benefits of the substance, he omitted the diet and official medicaments and used only propolis.

His success was rapid and of precise, measurable value. Using normal methods of treatment, 10 per cent of patients obtained relief from pain within three days. In the same time span, 70 per cent of patients taking propolis experienced the same relief. Of the former group, 25 per cent were relieved from pain by the seventh day; for the group on propolis the percentage was 75. Examination by X-ray revealed that 30 per cent of the first group and 60 per cent of the propolis group were healthy.

Ultimately the disease recurred in a number of patients and was treated operatively in 15 per cent of cases from the control group, but only 5 per cent of the propolis group.

At the end of the test, Dr Feiks made the convincing statement that the use of propolis shortens the length of treatment, rapidly diminishes pain, that it increases the number of effective cures, and reduces the necessity for later surgical treatment.

Of course, Dr Feiks was only researching the effects of propolis on the *healing* of ulcers. Ulcers have a number of causes – either dietary, arising within the organism or in the surrounding environment – and neither propolis nor the bees have the power to defeat the origins of this disease. Man alone can treat the sources of disease, and only if he has enough will-power and strength. Fortunately, however, the use of propolis at the critical moment for both patient and disease may ensure a successful and lasting cure.

Certainly the value of propolis may be confirmed by a modest, retiring old lady, of exactly eighty-one years of age who, after twelve years of torture with a stomach ulcer, came to Dr Feiks. For twelve years doctors had been convinced that only surgery would help her, and for the entire twelve years they had been afraid to perform that operation. For they very well knew that her heart was not strong and that she would probably not survive the operation.

Dr Feiks suggested that she take propolis and she naturally agreed. After six weeks the X-rays revealed that the treatment had been completely successful. A year later the ulcer had not re-opened and in the second and third years following they found that the ulcer was beautifully healed. In the fourth year the old lady died unexpectedly. No, not from a stomach ulcer, but from heart failure. Her heart had handed in its notice; finally everyone must die.

Because we know that the results of X-rays are not always reliable, final answers to all questions and doubts must be obtained at a time when they are of interest only to science – after death, by autopsy. In the stomach of the old lady the pathologist discovered, as the X-rays had sixteen years earlier, that she had indeed had an ulcer; but he also discovered that instead of the ulcer there remained only a scar, healed and completely closed.

CHAPTER EIGHT

A NATURAL ANTIBIOTIC

'We have known about antibiotics for some thirty years, during which time they have saved millions of human lives. Surgery has been known to mankind for thousands of years and it too has saved millions of lives.

'There are many differences between antibiotics and surgery but the most important distinction, I think, is this. If a person feels a pain in his stomach, or his head aches, or anything else, he does not go first to a surgeon (though there are exceptions, especially with accident cases). Either he, or a doctor, will begin with other means of treatment: a few days in bed, a herb tea, a change of diet, relaxation, different tablets or injections. Only when they are sure there is no alternative does the surgeon's scalpel get a turn. On the other hand, it frequently happens that someone with a pain in his stomach or a headache will leave out the rest, change of diet and the various other simple remedies and straight away take extreme measures – hundreds, thousands, millions of units of penicillin, streptomycin and who knows what other antibiotics.

'It is obviously true that we are too frequently using too

many antibiotics, in spite of the fact that we are especially warned against the harmful consequences of their use in the oral cavity. On the one hand they should be avoided in the treatment of various diseases of the membranes of the oral cavity, but on the other we cannot avoid the use of antibiotics and corticosteroids because we have no alternative method of treatment. We continue to turn the malevolent wheel from which we have no escape, other than the discovery of a new cure!'

Dr Perushek paused for a moment and glanced at his students, all of whom were carefully listening to his dissertation. They all knew that medical science finds itself in the difficult situation of having to use medicaments about which it has doubts and, within a year or two, they too would have to decide which medicines would be more beneficial than harmful and whether their use was really necessary. But at that moment they were not doctors, merely students, and could safely leave the lecturer to wrestle with the malevolent circle of antibiotics. For once, however, he surprised them, ordering them to observe some grains which he shook onto the table.

'Patients were the first to bring propolis to our attention,' calmly continued Professor Dr Milan Perushek, head of the Department of Oral Diseases at the stomatological clinic in Ljubljana. 'Patients told us that they had obtained propolis from acquaintances, from beekeepers, that they had been using it and that their teeth were very much strengthened. They had noticed that there were no more secretions from periodontal pockets in the gums, where the flesh had receded, or among the roots of their teeth, that gums ceased to bleed, and also that propolis acted very quickly against tonsilitis and bronchitis!'

The doctor smiled roguishly. With his warm, friendly eyes he absorbed the embarrassment and surprise in his students faces, for he could guess their thoughts. From their point of view, being as old as he was and having the profession he had, he was already ossified, had already embraced all the possible thoughts and truths: to trust all that was unproven, to destroy all that was traditional, that was their task and *their* right. Had the school of medical science *really* discovered something new?

'We began by using propolis in an alcohol solution,' Dr Perushek explained, 'and we are now examining the effect in two ways: periodontopathically and with the primary and secondary diseases of the oral membranes. On the whole we are satisfied with the results. We can ascribe a very important role to propolis because of its valuable effect in rapidly curing diseases of the oral membranes and also because it can be prescribed instead of the too frequent, inexpedient and sometimes totally harmful, use of antibiotics.'

PROPOLIS TESTS
He spoke for an hour of the propolis tests and everything he said was new to his students. He told them it was invaluable in the case of aphthae, the ulcers which appear in the membranes of the oral cavity and which are extremely painful. Stomatitis, one of the most frequently occurring diseases, could not be treated since available medicaments were washed away by saliva before they had a chance to act. Treatment with corticosteroids, antibiotics, or gammaglobulin was not particularly successful and for this reason the clinic began using propolis. After the first or second treatment patients felt better: the sores on the membranes were covered with a thin layer of propolis, not-withstanding the flow of saliva;

the inflamed area round each ulcer was reduced as also was the pain, allowing patients to eat normally. The ulcers healed completely and rapidly, particularly if the patient had used propolis from the onset of the disease.

With various periodontopathic diseases, propolis was introduced as a very successful medicament. Gums slowly returned to a normal colour, becoming firm, and bleeding all but ceased. Where the flesh had already receded from the teeth, and the periodontal pockets had been scraped, propolis promoted healing and the adhesion of new tissue to the dental cement. After the surgical treatment of gums, it was affirmed that the use of propolis, instead of sulphanilamides or antibiotics, promoted rapid healing of the injured flesh.

Dr Perushek also used propolis in cases which had been seemingly hopeless, for instance in treating a girl who had been suffering from chronic inflammation of the gums. Her gums were permanently bright red, the bone had begun to decay, her teeth were loose and there was, all in all, a serious danger that the girl would lose them. Doctors had tried everything. Above all they had tried to uncover the cause of the disease, at first in her oral cavity alone and then elsewhere in her body, but the examinations remained unsuccessful.

The girl was growing up, becoming aware of how serious the problem was, from time to time crying about her inflamed gums. Her mind was obsessed with how terrible it would be to lose all her teeth at only sixteen.

She now calls frequently at the clinic and daily rinses her mouth with propolis. The treatment is not yet complete and who knows if it ever will be. Nevertheless all the teeth remain in her jaw and the despair in her eyes is slowly disappearing.

'We are using propolis on a skin virus called herpes,'

56

the professor announced to his students. 'The disease stomatitis herpetica is chiefly a disease of children and until now treatment has been only symptomatic and preventive of the secondary infection. By using propolis patients soon feel better and are able to enjoy eating, which had previously been their most difficult problem. Obvious and rapid results were also obtained in the treatment of herpes of the lip.'

He told them of a young man of twenty-six who had been accepted at the clinic.

'Two and a half years earlier he had received radiation treatment for a cancer of the throat glands of which some side-effects remained; his oral membranes were erythematous, inelastic and sensitive; he produced too little saliva and it was too thick; the patient had a burning taste in his mouth and he could swallow food only with the utmost difficulty. After discussion with the Oncological Institute we gave him Hexoral, without any satisfactory improvement. We decided on a 2 per cent propolis ointment. After four days the patient felt better and from objective observation also seemed improved; the membranes returned to a more normal colour, saliva increased in quantity and assumed a better viscosity. The patient is still under our observation.'

Dr Perushek told the students many many other things, and they listened attentively, the whole room filled with awe at what the lecturer was saying. Then, as sometimes happens, everything changed momentarily, some irresistible force took over and they burst out laughing. Yes, real uproarious laughter, so that one might think he would be angry, but finally he also began to laugh with the others.

Had the lecturer made a mistake? Had his words become confused during his description of an injury to a woman's tongue? Perhaps there was some hidden joke?

He was laughing himself although there was really nothing funny. Then, when the students had settled down, he started to explain, shrugging his shoulders and fixing them with a cheerful glance:

'Really, they brought her in with an injured tongue; I didn't believe it myself. Look, have you ever tried to hammer a lid onto a box and discovered that you haven't enough hands? Probably you too put the spare nails in your mouth for a moment or two. She was hurrying to tidy up after the children and put into her mouth a wire which was attached to an electric train. She was badly burnt and propolis helped her, chasing away the pain and healing the damage, just as with all other injuries to the oral cavity.'

Then, realizing that his lecture time had run out, Dr Perushek drew his talk to a close with these words: 'Propolis is a medicine which we can get from every beekeeper. People have often used it of their own accord and they are certain that it will help them, although it is not, of course, a means of treating every disease. If it was expected to cure every illness there would be much disappointment and people would lose their faith in a substance which, in the right place and at the right time, is extremely beneficial. Finally, you must not forget to warn patients of one permanent and indisputable fact: the maintenance of a healthy oral cavity begins with the right care, and before other medicaments it is necessary to use a good toothbrush and water!'

CHAPTER NINE

A CURE FOR CANCER?

He had been alive for fifty years and did not have any idea what it was like to be ill. He was surprised when someone said he was ill; he knew only about working. It had always been the same, at home, at school and as a specialist in several foreign countries, for work and people he always found enough time – for himself and his health, never enough. He was satisfied that would take care of itself.

And then it happened, that thing which Rudy had never once anticipated and which certainly must never occur to hinder the fruition of his latest plans. Slowly but surely, however, disease ate away at his inexhaustible capacity for work. In the beginning he hid it even from himself, and when he was finally forced to accept the facts he betrayed himself to no one. He went on as if nothing had happened, working as usual, although it became increasingly difficult. After fifty years he had come to know illness, but he fought it off, yielding only slowly, step by step, until eventually others also noticed it.

The first warning was the arrival of terrible, throbbing pains, accompanied by cramps. Rudy's digestion slowly began to fail him and every day he suffered from mucous secretions, among which he noticed blood.

The doctors' examinations were especially tedious for him and it seemed that everyone was trying to drag him away from his work. It was unbearable to be away from work and to have to lie in hospital. Finally they diagnosed *colitis ulcerosa* and discharged him with a vast supply of medicines and instructions to follow a strict diet.

Once he had returned to work, Rudy often dropped in to see me on his way from the railway station. At first I always offered him something to eat and drink, then I stopped asking and he looked after himself in the kitchen. Once he asked for a cup of tea, another time for camomile, both times without sugar. From a briefcase in which people usually carry papers, he would take something wrapped in foil, a piece of stale bread, which he would eat slowly crumb by crumb, washing it down with tea. I knew it must be difficult for him to become accustomed to such a diet and that I would only aggravate his difficulties if I helped myself to anything better, so each time I drank tea with him and made myself a proper meal when he had gone.

As a main meal he would eat plain boiled rice, with perhaps some boiled vegetables, especially boiled carrots without butter. For a change he would have boiled potatoes and carrots, again without butter, and we all knew that the third menu was rice purée. That was all, and all there had been for four years.

Ah yes, then there were the medicines, which he ate with the rice and potatoes so frequently that taking his medicine became almost an essential part of his eating. I still don't know what was prescribed for him; probably everything that could be found in our pharmacies and other remedies which had been sent him by friends from outside Jugoslavia.

They decided to see if a new drug from Sweden would help him. He tried it and, although it seemed to him that the pain became more bearable, his stomach completely ceased functioning. At the hospital where he was taken, they decided that he could not stand the tablets and they they would have to try an alternative treatment, if one could be found. And a change of diet; *polenta* (maize porridge), as well as rice purée and potatoes!

CANCER THREAT

Someone told me that Rudy had taken a turn for the worse and was back in hospital, then threw in the information that an acquaintance, Joseph, had died a few days earlier, also from cancer. That 'also' sounded strangely suspicious to me, as if it was his own diagnosis on our friend Rudy: he was certainly still alive, but he was in a bad way.

In the hospital there were the same thoughts and fears badly concealed in glances, scarcely veiled by the unfinished words of the doctor, and apparent also in the eyes of the patient. His feverish uncertainty, greyish-yellow skin, sunken face, his contrivedly friendly and cheerful greeting when I visited him, all indicated the same thing.

He told me of his latest plans, for he had always been full of new ideas. This one, however, was rather overworked, as tired as Rudy himself. From his manner and conversation he was trying to convince me that he was still strong but I felt a growing shadow of doubt and became convinced that everything was completely different. By the time I left the hospital I finally understood the unspoken message that Rudy had cancer.

Later, when they sent him home from hospital, I visited

him again with two other friends. We had decided that we must visit him, even though it made us feel uneasy. Apparently he guessed what our visit meant, although we tried to think up a convincing enough reason for visiting him; we did not want him to think that we had come too early to his funeral.

As before, he gave us first a shot of real, home-made plum brandy, then a glass of dry farmhouse wine from the hills of Haloze, and his good wife brought a whole dish of delicacies to the table. We ate and drank, talking all the while with perhaps exaggerated cheerfulness and certainly with unnecessary volume. He listened to us but didn't want to look at us; he was busy making work for himself – dashing down to the cellar, rummaging through the telephone directory, and even finishing a job in the garden.

When he came back, I went straight to the point. Putting down my knife and fork, although my plate was still full, pushing away my glass, I took a bottle from the breast pocket of my jacket and showed it to him.

'Rudy, try this. If the doctors and chemists can't help you maybe the bees can!'

'Give it to me, even if it's poison,' he said. 'As I am now I might just as well not be alive.'

A GLEAM OF HOPE

We saw, all three of us, and neither did it escape the notice of Rudy's wife, how a small flicker of hope leapt into his eyes and how eagerly he stretched out a hand for the bottle. 'Ten or fifteen drops in a little water,' I advised him, as the specialist had told me. 'Dr Kern says that will be enough! Three times a day, half an hour before meals.'

He poured some water into a small glass and started to add the liquid propolis from a dropper. He counted the drops with pursed lips and worried eyes, his hand trembling slightly.

As soon as they came in contact with the water, the drops vanished, changing the liquid to a cloudy, milky white colour. Rudy shook the glass and lifted it to the light, examining it as if it were the finest wine. Slowly and carefully he drank it, afraid it might all be a dream. Then he sat down and we three watched him as if at any moment something might occur. Nothing did, except that Rudy no longer behaved as if he were trying to escape from us, or from himself, but there was still an air of expectancy in the quiet room.

We talked again for a long time, about anything at all, just to pass the time and to prevent us from having to leave. Our host and hostess looked after their guests very well, there being in the cellar more than enough of the pleasant wine from Haloze.

Then, maybe an hour later, Rudy broke into our discussion and with wide eyes exclaimed: 'Boys, the pains have stopped!'

Some days later he even more excitedly announced on the telephone: 'Still no pains, no cramps, no blood! Listen, if it's true, it'll be a real miracle!'

And later still: 'I've eaten a steak, a whole steak, and I drank half a litre of wine!'

After that he requested: 'Please send me another bottle of propolis. The first is finished.'

JOYFUL REUNION

Six weeks passed, maybe a day or two more, but certainly it was less than seven weeks. We were again gathered at Rudy's farmhouse, all of us who had been there those few weeks earlier. But no one felt embarrassed this time, nobody was worried anymore that one of us was condemned to an early grave; we had not come to observe the passing away of a life, but to welcome in a second life which was just beginning.

Rudy informed us that he had put on a whole seven kilos since we had last been to see him. This much he told us and the rest we were able to see for ourselves; healthy pink cheeks, the same enthusiastic, self-confident look in his eyes, decisive movements and quick, firm footsteps.

Above all, he overflowed with plans and ideas, had great hopes that he would be able to work again, to catch up on the past seven years and wipe them from his life as if they had never existed.

CHAPTER TEN

THE BACTERIOLOGICAL BATTLEFIELD

Professor Mihael Likar, who has only been briefly mentioned until now, was a young man, seemingly too young to have accomplished all that he in fact had. The results of much of his work in basic microbiology had been reported in the most respected microbiological journals thoughout the world; he had published a number of specialized books; had worked at the Alexander Fleming Institute for penicillin research in London; he was the first to isolate the virus of Central European meningitis which is transferred by ticks; and the results of his work were published in the Bulletin of the World Health Organization. By all rights he should have been a much older man, with slightly tired eyes and halting gait, ready for an honourable retirement, satisfied with his life's work, and content to leave whatever remained.

He was, however, still a young man, this bacteriologist and virologist from the Institute of Microbiology at the University of Ljubljana's Medical Faculty. He was indifferent to those rules of life which should have ordered his existence but those rules which he made for himself could not be faulted by anyone.

Being as he was, he listened eagerly to his colleagues, giving his undivided attention to their account of a natural substance which, supposedly, possessed remedial properties to heal injuries and relieve inflammation, both of which were special fields of interest within the Institute.

A microbiological institute is very much a world of its own, a world in which each person has his own precisely defined areas of interest but a common enemy – microbes. It is at the same time a place of friendly co-operation between people and relentless battle against the merciless attack of an enemy which is innumerable and invisible to the naked eye.

Professor Likar weighed the evidence. Propolis, a product of the beehive. Why not? It sounded very interesting and perhaps had invaluable properties. But then there was already a long line of research workers who had been convinced that they had discovered natural medicinal substances, from which they had obtained nothing useful and which had caused them only embarrassment.

Professor Likar listened to everything. He took off his coat to be more comfortable, undid his tie and the top buttons of his shirt, lit his pipe, and made some strong Turkish coffee on the gas cooker in the laboratory.

Yes, propolis, why not? Especially if he could produce for the Institute a new, more successful drug, a new ally in the fight against microbes.

He went on listening for a long time and after the discussion he began to read – reports from biologists, chemists and doctors which made modest claims for propolis. The reports were interesting but not full enough. The Institute, with more than ten years experience researching hundreds of chemical substances and their effects on micro-organisms, could conduct a much fuller examination.

After he had thought for a while, Likar went to talk with another colleague and asked him what he knew about propolis. This man could not give any details but he maintained nevertheless that it had been subjected to examination and nothing valuable had been discovered. Propolis had nothing to do with science and as a research project was certainly not worth the effort.

The virologist laughed quietly to himself. Certainly that was the opinion of official medical science, born perhaps of slight jealousy. But those with the creative spirit need a challenge, for to be successful there, is all the more wonderful. Propolis was still very much in the dark world of the unknown and Professor Likar was a restless, inquisitive seeker of new truths; the man was made for the substance and the substance for the man!

SEEKING THE TRUTH

Thus propolis strayed onto the battlefield at the Institute, where protective substances within the cells fight for life or death with micro-organisms. It was introduced into bottles and test tubes, into chicken embryos and growing cultures, and was examined under microscopes.

Then propolis had to show the Institute what it was capable of doing, what in fact it had been doing for more than a million years. There was one more test it had to undergo to prove itself for all time to the whole world.

Among the first victims in the trials on living organisms and bacteriological cultures were types of staphlococci and streptococci. After many unsuccessful attempts with various chemical substances, propolis was in the end the first to inhibit the growth and activity of the microbe proteus; the results of this meeting with the influenza virus were really astonishing.

In ten years of experimenting on that virus with some hundreds of chemical substances, only two or three produced even minor activity. To all the rest the virus remained insensitive. The only really successful agent remains the substance amantadin, first synthesized in Switzerland thirty years ago by Jugoslavian-born Professor Dr Vladimir Prelog, who received the Nobel Prize in 1975.

Propolis produced an extremely active response from the virus. In the Institute they repeated the experiments many times to exclude all possibility of mistakes and were still highly gratified by the results.

After the first confirmation Professor Likar was able to write cautiously: 'The substance exhibits antimicrobial properties and would withstand the most detailed examination.'

In the Institute they prepared a strategic plan of action. They chose a representative of the enemy forces, the most typical and the most frequently manifest microbe, and Professor Likar also looked about for an ally. He decided on one of the youngest workers, 25-year-old Bratko Filipich. His choice was the result of the most careful consideration, and more than justified. For the young scientist lived only for microbiology, a choice he had made earlier still at high school.

In the Institute Filipich was researching interferons, especially albumin, from which the organism creates for itself a defensive weapon against the origins of various diseases. He had shown that the receptors of the interferon on the surface of the cells of the human organism are the same as those on which the hormones of the adrenal gland, cortisone, are fixed.

The announcement of this discovery was sent to the specialist bulletin *Interferon Scientific Memoranda* in the United States of America and a little later they received from the editor-in-chief the news that the article would be published in the next issue of the journal, together with his sincere congratulations on the discovery.

But before all this happened something else occurred.

SYNTHETIC PROPOLIS

So that the task of testing propolis would not be too easy, the researchers needed a control substance for their experiments and instructed their chemists to prepare an artificial propolis. The chemists gathered together resins and balms, added other substances, mixed and kneaded it all together, and produced something which in colour, smell, rigidity and consistency, in taste and in all other properties was indistinguishable from propolis. Only the chemists knew which samples were real; the microbiologists must not know.

CROSSING THE BATTLE–FRONT

In a bacterial culture they began to cultivate various microbes, to which they then added the samples of propolis. As thirty years earlier Professor Fleming had noticed that a fungus in a Petri dish inhibited the growth of bacteria, thus heralding in the era of antibiotics, so at the Institute they ascertained that the action of propolis followed a similar course.

The results were entered on a special table. At first they experimented with a 10 per cent solution which they later diluted in the proportions of 1:2, 1:4, 1:8, and 1:16. They arranged the microbes on a horizontal line and on the vertical they marked the different samples of diluted propolis. Then they made a long perpendicular line of crosses, like the crosses in a graveyard in memory of the dead, except that these crosses indicated the strength of propolis and the hopes of human life. One cross whenever propolis retarded the growth of the microbes, two if the activity was strong, and three whenever it was extremely successful.

There were many microbes on the table but quite a lot more crosses.

The microbe which causes diphtheria, *Corynebacterium diphtheriae*, was defeated by the first sample, which won two crosses. This is perhaps not so important today, since all children are now immunized against diphtheria and even people who do contract the disease are successfully treated; nevertheless this is not always the case. Only a few years ago we buried a friend who had suffocated from a throat blockage caused by diphtheria because there had not been a doctor available to open his trachea; and in the winter of 1975 in Gelsenkirchen in West Germany four children died from this disease.

Propolis earned three crosses for the defeat of *Salmonella paratyphi B*, the cause of paratyphus, although there are other successful drugs against this microbe; the same may be said of *Listeria monocytogenes* which, along with others, is the cause of infectious inflammation of the membranes of the brain.

There were crosses beside the most stubborn opponent, against which antibiotics are on the whole no longer effective, proteus, or *Pseudomonas aeruginosa*, which may be blamed for a number of unpleasant and troublesome disturbances of the digestive system. And more crosses and still more crosses until the table was almost covered.

Perhaps the happiest result was with staphylococci. *Staphylococus aureus*, for instance, we meet everywhere – in infections and painful abscesses on and under the skin, in the skin inflammations of children, in osteomyelitis, periostitis, in infections and inflammations of the lungs, kidneys, and the brain, in infections of the middle ear, eyes, and in meningitis. It was present during the epidemic of Asian 'flu in the late 1950s, was responsible for the deaths of babies in hospital by causing an infection in the milk glands of nursing mothers. *Staphylococus aureus* is quite at home in our oral cavities, throat and oesophagus, where it causes a variety of infections and is present in many instances of food poisoning. It is a killer, an enemy of our good health, possibly the worst of all the bacteria and, unfortunately, the one which has a particularly lethal property. It is extremely resistant, unusually stubborn, and not the least sensitive. Not only is it not inhibited by drugs but it becomes even more virulent when it comes in contact with a medicament, frequently mounting a counter-attack and destroying that which should help us. The rout began with penicillin, and other antibiotics have been even less successful.

For this reason the crosses, the long line of crosses which propolis earned here, either on its own or in combination with a honey, were perhaps the most precious. They indicated an unexpected victory, signified many less crosses in the graveyard, and represented the saving of thousands of human beings from suffering and illness. Professor Likar and his young assistant were satisfied.

On one level of the distribution table, however, they were surprised at the lack of crosses, the line was empty or showed only a few solitary crosses. Why should one of all the samples have failed?

The answer was simple. Propolis would have lost its validity if that one line had not remained empty – if the artificial propolis had produced the same effects as the medicinal propolis!

THE POWER OF THE BEES

Therefore the experiments at the Microbiological Institute not only demonstrated and confirmed the value of propolis above all other antimicrobial substances, but it also showed that without the bees there can be no propolis.

If research workers had the ability, ingenuity, enough perseverence and time to follow the bee on its flight, they could collect everything which the bees collect on their flights and discover the recipe for propolis. Would it be successful though?

Perhaps it could earn a few isolated crosses on the distribution table, nothing more, for without bees there is no propolis and never can be. It is not merely a collection from various plants which have medicinal properties but must contain also part of the very bee itself, the secretions from its glands, without which the collection of balsams, resins, and pollen remains incomplete, as was the artificial propolis.

The results from using different samples also proved one other point. Samples of propolis gathered during changing seasons and from different sources varied quite markedly. Quite disparate effects were gained by using propolis from an alpine source in comparison with samples from, for instance, the Panonian plains. There were significant differences between propolis gathered on the Adriatic Coast and that gathered from the plateaus of the Dinara Mountains.

If we want to use propolis as a medicine and to obtain the widest possible benefit from it, the crop must be collected from early spring to late autumn, from beehives all over the country. Then it would be possible to say that we had achieved 'wide-spectrum' propolis.

PROPOLIS MEETS THE VIRUSES
Now let us go back to the Microbiological Institute in the Medical Faculty of the University of Ljubljana.

When the bacterial front line had been broken and defeated propolis met with the viruses.

Here it fought not alone but supported by almost all the other bee products. From the beehive, which is both the oldest and the most modern pharmacy, researchers took the following: honey, the most complete of all nutritious substances and for thousands of years a medicament; pollen which assures the growth and continuing existence of plants; the mysterious royal jelly which is capable of producing from the larva not a worker but a queen; and of course propolis, probably one of the most precious substances available for the promoting of human health.

The experiments were not carried out this time in artificial bacteriological cultures but on the living organism of an embryo in the process of maturing. Microbiologist Bratko Filipich chose to immunize with two substances chicken embryos at the eleventh day of their incubation period in the egg, already half way to maturity. The first substance was one of the most dangerous, a representative of the virus group, the virus of influenza A; and either simultaneously or a little later, the second, not a destructive but a protective and health giving agent, one of the preparations containing royal jelly and propolis.

By inhibiting the growth of the embryo or terminating its life propolis would show whether it had any toxic properties, whether or not it was poisonous to the organism. But the embryos remained and continued to grow as normal, proving that propolis was not toxic.

Above all propolis had to prove its strength against the influenza virus.

At 37 degrees Centigrade (98.6°F) they immunized the embryos with the required dosage of the preparation, in the proportion of 1:20, and after forty-eight hours took control observations. They ascertained that the honey preparation very strongly inhibited the virus; in professional terms, the titer haemagglutination was 1:2. The second series of tests, using the preparation in the proportion of 1:100, produced the same results, the numerical value remaining unchanged.

Another series used much smaller proportions of propolis than in the second series, namely 1:10,000, and the preparation still produced marked results although the titer haemagglutination was noticeably smaller, 1:4.

They were statisfied with these results but decided that it was easy enough to do one more test – a ratio of 1:100,000! The result still the same, still numerically 1:4! Such a glorious victory and on such a courageously defended frontier!

Yet Bratko Filipich paced the floor of the Microbiological Institute, his head down and his hands hanging loosely at his side. He was muttering quietly to himself, shaking his head, and thinking hard. What could be wrong, where had he missed the error, where had he gone astray? If only he could trust one of his colleages with his grave doubts, for it was obvious that the results could not possibly be true.

Professor Likar noticed that there was something bothering his young research worker and cautiously and tactfully he asked what was the matter.

'I don't know, only it seems impossible to me that the tests can be accurate,' he lamented. Then they went through everything together, examined everything, recapitulated the whole thing so that they could be absolutely certain that it was true.

And it was, in spite of the fact that it would be highly inconvenient to use the royal jelly and propolis in the honey preparation in such small proportions, since the former constituted only 1.5 per cent of the honey, the latter a mere 1 per cent. A combination of both effective substances had retarded the growth of the virus influenza A in the ratio of 1:4,000,000 (1:4 million).

Only the bee products, royal jelly and propolis, and interferon have proved to be successful in the battle against viruses.

CHAPTER ELEVEN

THE MEDICINE OF TOMORROW

In Bratislava on that great river, the Danube (which is not blue or crystal clear but greyish-brown and hopelessly muddy), halfway between the old part of the city, where once Hungarian Kings were crowned, and the factories of the modern city, a meeting of scientists from eleven different countries was taking place. They met to talk about the future, about the medicine of tomorrow, as they decided to call it. It was a meeting of doctors, veterinarians, pharmacists, chemists, biologists and microbiologists or, to put it officially: *The Second International Symposium on Propolis, Bratislava, 1976.*

The medicine of tomorrow can come not from today but can already be several million years old! This is a long time in human terms but much less for bees, for bees existed long before there was any trace of human life and even a long time before they began to manufacture propolis.

So long as bees were the same as other similar insects, like wasps, they did not need propolis. They did not worry about how to survive the cold winters; from year to year all died, only the fertilized queen bee surviving the winter hidden away in hibernation in some sheltered place. When the warmer weather came again each year she would awaken and start the life cycle all over again. She was the only link between the past and the future, the only witness to the past.

When the bees began a new era of communal living, when the whole colony had to survive with the queen, they had to make many innovations, among them the 'invention' of propolis. In the interest of an organized society and self-preservation they needed a medicine which would successfully protect them against different illnesses; thus the beehive became the first and oldest drug factory.

For mankind, however, propolis is without a past, for we are only now starting to learn about it and in learning have become convinced that in propolis we have indeed discovered the medicine of the future.

NEW EVIDENCE
The symposium on propolis consisted of some sixty reports on its value in mending broken bones, speeding up cell growth, curing diseases of mucous membranes, skin, high blood pressure, and various other conditions.

Active, serious, but always good humoured, Dr Chizmarik from the University of Bratislava was once again the main organizer of the meeting and he was proud to report that science had been able to analyze more than half of the components of propolis. Only three and a half years earlier, at the first symposium, less than a third of the components had been isolated. This success for science was also a personal triumph, since he had contributed more than anyone else to the research programme.

A scientist from Halle in Germany had been trying to establish which of all the substances in propolis had the highest value, which was the most effective in the fight against microbes. Many times he thought he was on the brink of finding the answer. It would be of real value, since factories throughout the world would be able to use his discoveries to produce a medicine from the most useful substance. But it seemed that this would, after all, not be achieved for some time: to date research has not been able to surmount the unexpected difficulties which arose almost at the end of the research programme. Perhaps there is not just one substance in propolis which is more valuable than all the others; perhaps propolis exists only as a whole, and can only be produced by one factory in the entire world, the beehive!

There were many lectures, and many, many reports during the three days of the conference all relating the findings and knowledge of many people who had devoted years of their creative lives to propolis. Among the throng was Dr Kern, the man who discovered it through Rado Seifert who accidently cut the tip off his finger with some secateurs. That was a long time ago, and at innumerable meetings since he had learned many unexpected things about the remedial powers of propolis. He sat almost reverently in front of the screen in the hall, watching the changing pictures, the large, sometimes shocking colour photographs.

On the screen there first appeared an ear covering the whole screen. The outside of this enlarged ear was nicely hollowed and clear but in the middle a horribly unnatural growth appeared.

This was followed by another picture, again an ear, but not at all like the first ear, even if it was in fact the same one. With his capable hands, the surgeon had removed the ghastly wart. The danger was over, it had been cut down to the cartilage, leaving only the fresh wound. Left as it was the cartilage would receive no nourishment, would die and shrivel to a shapeless mass. For this reason the doctors would do a transplant, taking skin from another area, usually in the neighbourhood, so that the skin would take hold and regrow; the ear would be restored and only deep scarring would remain.

Then on the screen the same ear was shown again, the wound now considerably smaller although no skin graft had been performed. From all sides it was covered, right to the edges. Something unusual must have happened, for there is no literature which says this is possible without a transplant.

Finally, once more filling the screen, there was the ear. Where the open wound had been there was now skin, taut and clear, without any trace of scarring. Dr Kern stood by the screen, a pointer in his hand, and explained to the audience that he had frequently bathed the wound with propolis. There was the answer to the puzzle of the slides on the screen.

THE DEDICATED RESEARCHER
Afterwards there followed a discussion which was frequently interrupted by a young man with persistent questions.

He was a tall, well-built man who stooped when he talked, as if wanting to come closer to the person he was questioning. He looked composed, one could say confident, but at the same time a little child-like. At times he was almost unpleasant, for he was uncovering both good and bad aspects of the reports. He was sceptical of everything, wanted to check everything.

Eventually someone threatened to take revenge on

him, first on his own behalf and then publicly: 'You wait till your turn comes, I'll examine your conscience. You'll see, you'll slip up.'

But the young man went on questioning. He didn't really want to put anyone on the spot, only wanted to know more, to be able to check his own work against the knowledge of others.

Others also began to ask questions. They became more and more interested to know who this inquisitive young stranger was.

'A microbiologist? From Jugoslavia? Filipich, from Ljubljana? The report on the effect of propolis and royal jelly on viruses?'

Viruses are, of course, one of todays topics of conversation, not only Bratislava but the whole world over. Only two months previously scientists from eleven countries had held the third international conference on anti-viral substances in New York where they discussed the possibilities of finding a medicine which would stop the deadly advance of viral infections. They could deal with bacterial and fungal infections with antibiotics, but viral infections remained undefeated.

Every year millions of people are attacked by viruses which cause influenza, diseases of the liver, painful herpes and lay the foundation for the uncontrollable growth of cancer. In hospitals drugs are being tried which will one day be produced in factories, will be prescribed by doctors and will be on sale in pharmacies throughout the world. There may come the day when the usual prescription for influenza will not be merely aspirin, hot lemon juice and a trip to bed, because we know of nothing better. There may come the day when the unceasing battle between viruses and vaccines will be won, the battle in which vaccines are always one step behind viruses that can yearly change their properties, proving that they are not yet captured nor will be caught.

Only two months before the conference in New York, a young, inquisitive, almost child-like microbiologist modestly announced in Bratislava, 'We have discovered and are already producing a natural substance which has a retarding effect on the growth of the influenza virus.'

For many the report compiled by Bratko Filipich and his professor, Mihael Likar, was not very exciting – there were no dramatic revelations, only numbers and statistics, viruses and their cultures. Only the reasoning was dramatic, and the implication that we were coming to the era of victory over viruses, the moment which had previously lived only in the hopes of scientists.

More moving was the modest, but nevertheless self-confident, announcement:

'A natural substance which inhibits the growth of the influenza virus is here! It can be obtained without any prescription in every pharmacy in our country. From the big supermarkets if one doesn't want to go to a pharmacy!'

CHAPTER TWELVE

THE VIRUS IS VANQUISHED

Bratko Filipich had devoted himself only to the study of viruses. His first discoveries at the Institute of Microbiology had spurred him on to others. Once a person had started as he did, it becomes impossible to give up under any circumstances.

After his successes using propolis, Filipich was looking for new ways to test the substance and an interesting thought came to him.

What would happen if, instead of trying to copy nature or to succeed where nature itself had failed, a microbiologist were simply to listen attentively to nature's own knowledge and memory? What would happen if, in the fight against viruses, he collected all the substances which, though completely different in origin and function, have the same goal: to maintain life and to frustrate death?

What would be the combined anti-viral effect of royal jelly, propolis, and interferon? This would combine substances from two entirely different sources, two from a bee, weighing but a few grammes, the other from a rabbit weighing several kilograms; the first contributing to the battle a substance which he makes himself, the latter contributing a substance manufactured in the cells of his kidneys.

These substances were brought together in experiments using developing chicken embryos and in later experiments with new types of viruses. Still one more substance in the wide palette of tomorrow's medicine?

Filipich had courage enough to try the new experiments and luck did not desert him: the strange new substance, born of imagination, worked extremely well against the vesicular virus stomatitis. Which virus would be next?

The corneas of a hare's eyes were lined with small, almost imperceptable cuts, firstly only round the pupils, then radiating out in straight lines like beams. They had not occurred naturally, but had been deliberately and carefully cut by the research worker, so that the herpes virus could be implanted in them. The cornea is a layer of cells which provides a type of laboratory culture for viruses and, since it is part of a living animal, can show the degree of success of treatment should the undesirable infection be the result of natural causes. The virus would develop in these cuts, causing infection and damage until the research worker applied whatever substance he was using to restrict its growth. If the small scars remained as at the beginning and the growth of the infection abates, then the experiment would have proved that the test substance was stronger than the disease. The greater the number of cuts where the infection was forced to desist, the greater the strength of the medicament.

Three hours after implanting the virus the research worker coated the injured area with the anti-viral substance. He repeated the process after six hours, continuing thus for three days and three nights. This battle between virus and medicament gave rise to the following conclusion.

'Without doubt a combination of royal jelly, propolis, and interferon from the kidneys of a hare is victorious over the herpes virus of the cornea. One more triumph!'

Was this really the dawning of a new era in the fight for human health and survival? Had the time really come for victory over that dangerous enemy in the treacherous world of the virus?

Sad to say, the knowledge of the microbiologist was still limited to the enclosed circle within the laboratory, extending only to artificial cultures, chicken embryos, and the eyes of hares. From there to experimental treatment of patients there was still a long way to go. There were many difficulties to be overcome for propolis on the path to successful production – hundreds of samples, hundreds of analyses, tests and experiments, and a great deal of time. Final approval rested with the doctors, with the patients and with the maintenance or restoration of human health.

A STEP TOWARDS RECOGNITION

The first step was a small jar of honey containing a natural antimicrobial substance obtained from the bees; it was packaged in a pleasant, light yellow carton on which was written *Apikompleks*. That was only the beginning.

It was the doctors and patients who answered the question of what would happen when a virus met this natural substance, not in the foetus of a chicken or the cornea of a hare, but in the human organism. The first answer was short, a letter written in the form of a telegram: 'Herpetic eruption on lip first noticed Tuesday, one centimetre long. Ointment with propolis and royal jelly received one day later, Wednesday. Applied three times daily, first removing the old ointment from the lip before re-application. Eruption dried rapidly, by Sunday scab already dropped off. Best results were seen in the mornings. The ointment certainly helped me as no other medicament to date.'

FIGHTING 'FLU
The second answer came from Hajra and Izet, from Maria and Vera and many others. I must not forget that one of these is a doctor, Professor Dr Izet Osmanagic from Sarajevo, who organized the experiment. All the others were the girls from a nursing college.

That winter a serious epidemic of influenza attacked the town of Sarajevo. Professor Osmanagic explained to the students that this was the right time for an experiment.

In the six classes of the school they must organize a group of 63 students who, for approximately two months, would take a teaspoon of a natural preparation called Melbrosin propolis* every morning. The remaining 157 would not take it. Of 50 teachers, half would take the preparation and the doctors would follow the development of influenza in the two groups.

'Why can't I take it?' asked many of the girls, and the professor had to explain that in the interests of science they must be able to draw comparisons and that, in any case, there were not enough jars of the preparation.

To each of those who had been chosen he gave two yellow boxes with a pot of honey inside, and they then took a spoonful every day.

'Give me a bit, just to try,' asked one friend of another, but to no avail. Later, when she felt tired and sleepy, when she felt strange pains in her temples and her forehead felt hotter and hotter, she was still not given any.

'I would give you some,' the friend concluded, 'but I mustn't. The professor told us that would make the experiment valueless. If it's like this next year I'll recommend you for treatment, but this year you can't have any, in the name of science!'

The epidemic in Sarajevo spread, into the factories, schools and other places. Beds in hospitals and homes filled. Then, of course, it began to abate and, with the end of winter and the coming of the warm spring weather, it disappeared.

When the papers and statistics about the propolis experiment were examined they showed that of 157 students who were not given the propolis* 63, or 38.8 per cent, became ill; of 63 students who were given it 6, or 9 per cent, became ill.

All the students, the ones who remained healthy with propolis and the ones who were sick without it, gave their verdict. 'Yes, it really does protect you from influenza; Apikompleks is a great medicine!'

* Called Apikompleks in Jugoslavia.

CHAPTER THIRTEEN

HIGH HOPES FOR PROPOLIS

The tent beside the cliff was half-covered with snow by morningfl The two hen who had spent the night in its confined space wanted to move outside to meet the first rays of sunlight touching the mountain peaks, yet at the same time they were reluctant to leave the shelter of the canvas tent.

Legend maintained that under this mountain was the centre of the earth, where lay an incredibly beautiful, fantastically large lotus. The petals of the lotus were said to stretch to the four corners of the earth, so that every place in the world was connected with this spot. Yet, even if in legend, this mountain was the crossroads of the world, the camp seemed utterly isolated.

Up there everything depended on the courtage, the will and the strength of two men – Zvone and Joseph. On the second cordee they began to fight their way up the last part of the 2,500 metre cliff to repeat the victory of the first cordée, tying the ropes all the way to secure the descent of the men who had already reached the summit.

The mountaineers would probably say that they chose

Mount Trisul because in Jugoslavia they have a mountain with the name Triglav – a different word, certainly, but having the same meaning. But there was another reason which had some bearing on the decision. Trisul was the first mountain in the Himalayas attempted by a Jugoslavian expedition, sixteen years ago. That expedition conquered the peaks Trisul II and Trisul III but had neither the time nor good enough weather for Trisul I. The most crucial factor was the west wall, as yet unconquered and 2,500 metres high; years ago alpinists had examined it carefully and decided that it was probably unconquerable. That was why Trisul I was chosen in spite of the fact that our climbers had been higher. The challenge lay not in the attainment of mere height, but in the encounter with an unyielding, unconquerable cliff.

For my story Trisul I has a different significance: victory on this occasion meant also another first in the history of bees. Among the participants on the first climb over the west wall at the top of Trisul I was propolis.

After an almost sleepless night Zvone and Joseph collected together everything they would need for the journey to the summit. Before leaving they ate some of the contents of a small glass jar; it was Melbrosin propolis, for health and strength. It was a wonderful day and, although the gale was formidable in its strength, the summit was clothed in a rainbow of ice and crystal plumes, reaching almost to the sky. The climbers travelled through the snow storm along the ridge, their heavy feet sometimes sinking deeply into the fresh snow. Elsewhere the crampons bit with all their might into the ice, frustrating the efforts of the wind to snatch away the victory. Around them, reaching to the skyline, were the mountain chains and the jagged stumps of countless peaks; below them the thick, restless mass of fog hid the valley. But there was little time to admire all this beauty; the only thing was the task in hand, to defeat the cliff and reach the summit!

A little after 9 am they made it. On the very top of the mountain they planted a ski stock and tied to it their national flag. With cold fingers, which even three pairs of gloves could not protect well enough, they adjusted their sights and took pictures. They had no strength for hand-shaking, whistling, and other expressions of general joy, nor for any thoughts about the solemnity of the moment. They had a moment to feast their eyes on the scene, to fix in their memories the beauty of the country which is supposedly the centre of the world; then, with fire in their hearts and icicles on their beards and moustaches, they returned to camp.

In the tent Vanja and Janez, from the third or fourth cordée, had melted some snow and mixed a few spoonsful of honey into the warm water, making the most highly appreciated drink in the Himalayas. The victorious party descended the ropes for another 350 metres to warmth and luxurious rest.

SUCCESS AT THE SUMMIT

The expedition had not finished its tasks yet, for they had to clean the mountainside, a thing which tourists the world over very often forget to do. And they had to carry on an experiment of an unusual sort – to test what would happen to certain products from a beehive at such a height where the sunbeams are richer and stronger than elsewhere, where a load may either freeze in a knapsack or fry in the burning crevasses.

Later, in the laboratory, they determined that the substance from the beehive had withstood these difficulties unusually well. Of their benefits to the alpinists, the doctor of the expedition, Borut Pirc, wrote, 'The whole time members of the team consumed large quantities of honey. It proved to be an excellent source of nourishment because of its ability to satisfy the enormous calorie needs of alpinists at great heights.'

The leader of the expedition, experienced alpinist Tony Sazonov, related that for thirst and exhaustion they had found it most benficial to drink honey diluted in tepid water and that they had supplemented meals with honey and Melbrosin propolis when other food had run out.

One member of the team had fallen, receiving large bruises which had become infected; these had been bathed with propolis solution and had quickly cleared and healed.

Tony Sazonov talked willingly of the protective cream containing propolis and royal jelly. Comparing it with ointments taken on previous expeditions he concluded that this one was the best. To this fact he could give personal witness, since he had forgotten to put any protective cream on the exposed parts of his skin and had become quite sunburned. Not having the bee cream with him, he had tried several others; this was doubly painful, firstly from the sunburn and secondly from the cream on his cracked skin. Only back at camp, when he found and used the cream containing propolis, did it ease.

Of the samples of this cream Dr Pirc wrote. 'All members of the team were supplied with the cream; it has a pleasant smell, softens the skin, and successfully prevents sunburn.'

There were further convincing findings from the doctor. 'The team experienced no serious medical problems resulting from the use of a range of bee products. I would recommend their use in future as a preventative measure and these products should certainly not be excluded from the equipment of any such expedition.'

CHAPTER FOURTEEN

FULL CIRCLE

We were sitting again in front of Cene's beehives in Repnje, on the bench or on the ground. The bench was hard but the ground was even harder, for there was a drought – such a drought as we had not experienced for at least a hundred years. The soil was dry, the grass burnt, and the unripe fruit was falling to the ground. We glanced anxiously at the sky, which had been cloudless for days and days on end, and at the bees which flew off to the forests, returning laden with their sugary loads. The trees in the woods and the leaves of the fruit trees shone invitingly, so that the bees hardly knew where to fly to find the richest pastures.

We were silent, so as not to disturb the restless murmurings of the bees with unnecessary words. The pleasant afternoon mood was only disturbed by the noise of the drum which was turning a thick stream of honey into a half-filled container.

Later, tired, we stopped work and helped ourselves to a glass of schnapps from the bottle which had been leaning against the shady side of the tree to keep cool. The head of the house lit himself a cigarette and with great satisfaction took his first puff. We began to talk, as usual about matters of great importance: about crops and drought; about the honey, which after the previous bad year was plentiful this year; about buckwheat, which no one wanted to plant anymore; and then about mountains, the Himalayas, and the experience of our men with propolis, royal jelly and, of course, honey.

Someone said sagely,'This business on the Himalayas is not especially interesting; these mountaineers couldn't tell us much about the effect of propolis on diseases which they did not have.'

Cene, who was the most experienced and also the most purposeful of us all, as usual gave us his pronouncement. 'Friend, you must really be sick if you can't live without disease and medicines! Isn't it much better to be without disease, to remain healthy, with the bees' help of course!'

We all laughed while he surveyed the world around him with unusual seriousness.

He took no notice but went back into the house and returned carrying a bottle of wine. He poured it slowly into our glasses, then he mumbled, 'Maybe we're only a few today but we will be more and more every day, we who are sure that propolis is the medicine of tomorrow.'

The ruby red wine from the hills of Dolensko glittered in the raised glasses. Feeling the solemnity of the moment we stood up; looking through the crystal clear glasses at the sun, we thought of bees, of medicine from beehives, of ourselves, and of our fate. Then we touched our glasses together and gave the firm toast. 'To health, and to propolis!'